Mind Mapping for Women with Adult ADHD

Harnessing Your Brain's Full Potential and Empowering Your ADHD Journey

MARGOT PEARSON

Copyright © 2024

By MARGOT PEARSON

All rights reserved. No part of this publication may be reproduced, distributed, or transmitted in any form or by any means, including photocopying, recording, or other electronic or mechanical methods, without the prior written permission of the publisher, except in the case of brief quotations embodied in critical reviews and certain other noncommercial uses permitted by copyright law.

Table of Content

Copyright © 2024... 2
Table of Content.. 4
Introduction... 8
   Brief Introduction to the Book's Purpose.................. 8
   The Author's Journey with ADHD............................. 9
   Importance of Mind Mapping for Women with ADHD. 10
Understanding ADHD in Women............................... 12
   Overview of ADHD... 12
   Unique Challenges Faced by Women with ADHD.. 13
   The Power of Self-Acceptance and Self-Awareness.. 15
Part 1.. 18
Understanding Mind Mapping................................... 18
Chapter 1... 20
What is Mind Mapping?.. 20
   Definition and History... 20
   Benefits of Mind Mapping.. 21
Chapter 2... 26
How Mind Mapping Works....................................... 26
   The Science Behind Mind Mapping....................... 26
   How It Engages the ADHD Brain............................ 28
Chapter 3... 32
Tools and Techniques... 32
   Materials Needed for Mind Mapping...................... 32
   Various Mind Mapping Tools and Apps.................. 33
Part 2.. 40

Applying Mind Mapping in Everyday Life................40
Chapter 4..42
Personal Life...42
    Managing Daily Routines and Chores.................42
    Meal Planning and Grocery Shopping.................44
    Personal Goal Setting and Tracking.................46
Chapter 5..50
Professional Life..50
    Organizing Tasks and Projects at Work..............50
    Enhancing Creativity and Brainstorming.............52
    Time Management and Prioritization.................54
Chapter 6..58
Academic Pursuits...58
    Note-Taking and Studying Techniques................58
    Planning and Writing Essays or Reports.............60
    Preparing for Exams................................63
Part 3...68
Personal Development Through Mind Mapping......68
Chapter 7..70
Self-Care and Mindfulness................................70
    Using Mind Maps to Plan Self-Care Routines.........70
    Tracking Mood and Emotional Triggers...............74
Chapter 8..80
Stress Management..80
    Identifying Stressors and Coping Mechanisms........80
    Creating a Mind Map for Relaxation Techniques......83
Chapter 9..88
Building Healthy Relationships..........................88

    Mapping Out Communication Strategies............... 88
    Understanding Relationship Dynamics.................. 93
Part 4..**98**
Real-Life Success Stories..**98**
Chapter 10... **100**
Interviews with Women Who Use Mind Mapping.. 100
    Success Stories from Various Backgrounds......... 100
    How Mind Mapping Has Impacted Their Lives..... 108
Chapter 11..**110**
Personal Testimonies... **110**
    Anonymous Accounts and Tips from Readers...... 110
    Lessons Learned and Advice for Newcomers...... 115
Part 5..**118**
Getting Started with Your Own Mind Mapping Journey... **118**
Chapter 12... **120**
Step-by-Step Guide to Creating Your First Mind Map. 120
    Detailed instructions and examples...................... 120
    Tips for Overcoming Initial Hurdles....................... 123
Chapter 13... **128**
Developing a Mind Mapping Habit........................... **128**
    Strategies for Consistency and Motivation........... 128
    Setting Realistic Goals and Celebrating Progress 130
Conclusion.. **136**
    Recap and Encouragement.................................. 136
    Words of Encouragement and Empowerment...... 137
    Looking Forward.. 138

7

Introduction

Welcome Message

Welcome to "Mind Mapping for Women with Adult ADHD: Harnessing Your Brain's Full Potential and Empowering Your ADHD Journey." This book is a labor of love, born from my own experiences and struggles with ADHD. It is my sincere hope that through these pages, you will find the tools and inspiration needed to navigate your ADHD journey with confidence and clarity. Whether you are newly diagnosed or have been living with ADHD for years, this book aims to provide you with practical strategies, heartfelt encouragement, and a supportive community.

Brief Introduction to the Book's Purpose

The purpose of this book is to empower women with ADHD by introducing them to the powerful tool of mind mapping. Mind mapping is not just a technique; it is a transformative way of thinking that can help you organize your thoughts, manage your time, and achieve your goals. For women with ADHD, who often juggle multiple roles and responsibilities, mind mapping offers a structured yet flexible method to harness the full potential of our unique brains.

This book is designed to:

- Educate you about ADHD and its impact on women
- Explain the concept and benefits of mind mapping
- Provide practical applications of mind mapping in various aspects of life
- Share real-life success stories from women who have benefited from mind mapping
- Offer step-by-step guidance to help you start and maintain your mind mapping practice

By the end of this book, you will have a comprehensive understanding of how to use mind mapping to enhance your daily life, boost your productivity, and improve your emotional and mental well-being.

The Author's Journey with ADHD

I was diagnosed with ADHD in my mid-thirties, after years of feeling like I was constantly swimming against the tide. The diagnosis was both a relief and a revelation. It explained so much about my struggles with time management, organization, and focus. However, it also came with its own set of challenges. I had to learn how to navigate a world that wasn't designed for the way my brain worked.

My journey with ADHD has been one of self-discovery and growth. I experimented with various strategies and tools to manage my symptoms, and it was during this exploration that I stumbled upon mind mapping. Initially, it was just a fun and creative way to take notes, but soon, I realized its profound impact on my ability to organize thoughts, plan projects, and reduce overwhelm. Mind mapping became a cornerstone of my daily routine, helping me to harness the strengths of my ADHD brain rather than fighting against it.

Through this book, I want to share the insights and techniques that have helped me and many other women like me. My goal is to provide you with a resource that not only addresses the practical aspects of managing ADHD but also celebrates the creativity, resilience, and unique perspectives that come with it.

Importance of Mind Mapping for Women with ADHD

Women with ADHD often face unique challenges that can impact every aspect of their lives. These challenges can include managing household responsibilities, balancing work and family, dealing with societal expectations, and maintaining personal well-being.

Traditional organizational tools and methods often fall short, leading to frustration and a sense of inadequacy.

Mind mapping offers a dynamic and visually engaging way to tackle these challenges. Here's why mind mapping is particularly beneficial for women with ADHD:

1. **Visual Organization**: ADHD brains are often more visually oriented. Mind maps use colors, images, and spatial relationships to represent information, making it easier to process and recall.

2. **Flexible Structure**: Unlike linear lists and outlines, mind maps allow for non-linear thinking. This flexibility is perfect for the ADHD brain, which often jumps from idea to idea.

3. **Holistic View**: Mind maps provide a bird's-eye view of information, helping you see connections and relationships between different pieces of information. This holistic perspective can reduce feelings of overwhelm and increase clarity.

4. **Creative Expression**: Mind mapping taps into your creative side, making planning and organizing feel more like an art project than a

chore. This creative outlet can be both therapeutic and motivating.

5. **Customization**: Mind maps can be tailored to fit your personal style and needs. Whether you prefer digital tools or pen and paper, you can customize your mind maps to suit your preferences.

6. **Enhanced Focus**: The process of creating a mind map requires active engagement, which can help improve focus and concentration. It breaks down tasks into manageable chunks, making it easier to stay on track.

Understanding ADHD in Women

Overview of ADHD

Attention Deficit Hyperactivity Disorder (ADHD) is a neurodevelopmental disorder characterized by persistent patterns of inattention, hyperactivity, and impulsivity. While ADHD is commonly associated with children, it also affects millions of adults worldwide. ADHD manifests differently in each individual, and its symptoms can vary widely.

ADHD is often categorized into three types:

1. **Predominantly Inattentive Presentation**: Difficulty sustaining attention, following through on tasks, and organizing activities.
2. **Predominantly Hyperactive-Impulsive Presentation**: Hyperactivity, impulsiveness, and difficulty sitting still or waiting for turns.
3. **Combined Presentation**: A combination of inattentive and hyperactive-impulsive symptoms.

Unique Challenges Faced by Women with ADHD

Women with ADHD often face unique challenges that are not always recognized or understood. These challenges can impact various aspects of life, including personal relationships, career, and mental health. Some of the key challenges include:

1. **Late Diagnosis**: Many women are diagnosed with ADHD later in life, often after years of struggling with symptoms. This late

diagnosis can lead to feelings of frustration and missed opportunities for support.

2. **Masking and Compensatory Strategies**: Women with ADHD are often adept at masking their symptoms and developing compensatory strategies to cope with daily life. While these strategies can be effective, they can also be exhausting and lead to burnout.

3. **Societal Expectations**: Societal expectations and gender roles can add additional pressure on women with ADHD. The expectation to manage household responsibilities, childcare, and professional duties can be overwhelming, leading to increased stress and anxiety.

4. **Emotional Regulation**: Women with ADHD may experience heightened emotional sensitivity and difficulty regulating emotions. This can lead to mood swings, anxiety, and depression, which can further complicate their ADHD symptoms.

5. **Self-Esteem and Identity**: Struggling with ADHD symptoms and societal expectations can impact self-esteem and self-identity. Women may feel inadequate or constantly compare

themselves to others, leading to a negative self-image.

The Power of Self-Acceptance and Self-Awareness

Self-acceptance and self-awareness are crucial components in managing ADHD and living a fulfilling life. Embracing your ADHD and understanding how it affects you can empower you to develop strategies that work for your unique brain.

1. **Self-Acceptance**: Accepting your ADHD means recognizing that it is a part of who you are, and it does not define your worth or capabilities. It involves letting go of the idea of being "perfect" and instead focusing on your strengths and the unique qualities that ADHD brings to your life. Self-acceptance can reduce feelings of shame and guilt, and it allows you to approach challenges with a more positive and compassionate mindset.

2. **Self-Awareness**: Self-awareness involves understanding how ADHD affects your behavior, emotions, and interactions with the world. By becoming more aware of your triggers, strengths, and areas that need support, you can develop

effective strategies to manage your symptoms. Mind mapping is an excellent tool for increasing self-awareness, as it helps you visualize and organize your thoughts and emotions.

3. **Building a Support System**: Surrounding yourself with a supportive network of friends, family, and professionals can make a significant difference in managing ADHD. Support groups, therapy, and coaching can provide valuable insights, encouragement, and practical advice.

4. **Developing Coping Strategies**: With self-acceptance and self-awareness, you can develop personalized coping strategies that align with your strengths and needs. These strategies may include time management techniques, mindfulness practices, and creative outlets like mind mapping.

5. **Embracing Your Unique Brain**: ADHD comes with its own set of strengths, such as creativity, problem-solving skills, and the ability to think outside the box. Embracing these strengths and using tools like mind mapping can help you harness the full potential of your brain and turn challenges into opportunities for growth.

In this book, we will explore how mind mapping can be a powerful tool for increasing self-awareness, organizing your thoughts, and managing the unique challenges of ADHD. By combining self-acceptance with practical strategies, you can create a life that is not only manageable but also fulfilling and empowering.

Together, we will navigate the complexities of ADHD, celebrate the strengths it brings, and empower you to live your best life. Welcome to your journey of self-discovery and empowerment. Let's begin this adventure together.

Part 1
Understanding Mind Mapping

Chapter 1

What is Mind Mapping?

Definition and History

Mind mapping is a visual thinking tool that helps in organizing information, thoughts, and ideas in a structured yet flexible manner. It involves creating a diagram where a central concept or topic is placed in the middle, with related subtopics branching out radially. Each subtopic can further branch out into its own subtopics, forming a web of interconnected ideas. This method utilizes the brain's natural way of processing information through associations and visual imagery, making it easier to comprehend and remember complex concepts.

The concept of mind mapping was popularized by Tony Buzan, a British author and educational consultant, in the 1970s. Buzan's work was heavily influenced by his interest in the workings of the human brain and how it processes information. He observed that traditional note-taking methods were often linear and restrictive, failing to tap into the brain's full potential. Inspired by the brain's associative and imaginative capabilities,

Buzan developed mind mapping as a technique to enhance learning, memory, and creativity.

Although Buzan is widely recognized for formalizing mind mapping, the practice itself has roots in ancient history. Historical figures like Leonardo da Vinci and Albert Einstein employed similar methods to organize their thoughts and ideas visually. These early mind maps, although not referred to as such, were used to brainstorm, solve problems, and make sense of complex information.

Benefits of Mind Mapping

Mind mapping offers a multitude of benefits, especially for individuals with ADHD. These advantages make it a powerful tool for improving various aspects of life, from personal organization to professional productivity. Here are some of the key benefits:

1. **Enhanced Memory and Recall**
    - Mind maps engage multiple areas of the brain, making it easier to encode and retrieve information. The use of colors, images, and spatial arrangements helps create strong mental images, which are more memorable than traditional text-based notes. This can be particularly

beneficial for individuals with ADHD, who often struggle with memory and recall.

2. **Improved Organization**

    o Mind mapping provides a clear and intuitive way to organize information. By visually laying out ideas and their relationships, you can see both the big picture and the finer details simultaneously. This holistic view can help in understanding complex subjects and identifying connections between different pieces of information.

3. **Boosted Creativity**

    o The free-form and visual nature of mind mapping encourages creative thinking and exploration. Unlike linear note-taking, mind mapping allows you to jump between ideas, make new connections, and generate innovative solutions. This creative freedom can be particularly valuable for individuals with ADHD, who often have a rich imagination and unconventional thinking patterns.

4. **Increased Focus and Concentration**
    o Creating a mind map requires active engagement, which can help improve focus and concentration. The process of breaking down information into manageable chunks makes it easier to stay on task and reduces feelings of overwhelm. For individuals with ADHD, who may struggle with maintaining focus, this can be a game-changer.

5. **Efficient Problem Solving**
    o Mind maps facilitate a comprehensive view of problems and potential solutions. By visually mapping out the problem and its related factors, you can explore different angles and identify effective solutions more quickly. This can enhance decision-making and problem-solving skills, which are often areas of difficulty for those with ADHD.

6. **Enhanced Communication**
    o Mind maps can be an excellent tool for conveying complex information clearly and concisely. They provide a visual

summary that can be easily understood by others, making it easier to share ideas and collaborate. This can be particularly useful in team settings, where clear communication is essential.

7. **Personalized Learning**

    o Mind mapping allows you to tailor your note-taking and information processing methods to suit your individual learning style. Whether you prefer using visuals, keywords, or detailed notes, you can create mind maps that align with your preferences and needs. This personalization can make learning more effective and enjoyable.

8. **Stress Reduction**

    o The act of creating a mind map can be calming and therapeutic. It provides a sense of order and clarity, helping to reduce anxiety and stress. By visually organizing your thoughts, you can gain a better understanding of your priorities and tasks, making it easier to manage your time and responsibilities. For women with ADHD, who often juggle multiple roles and face constant pressures, this stress reduction can be incredibly beneficial.

Chapter 2

How Mind Mapping Works

The Science Behind Mind Mapping

Mind mapping is rooted in cognitive neuroscience, leveraging the brain's natural functions to enhance understanding, memory, and creativity. Here's a closer look at the science behind it:

1. **Brain Hemispheres**

    o The human brain is divided into two hemispheres: the left and right. The left hemisphere is associated with logical, analytical, and sequential thinking, while the right hemisphere is linked to creativity, imagination, and holistic thinking. Traditional note-taking methods often engage only the left hemisphere. In contrast, mind mapping activates both hemispheres, fostering a balanced and integrated approach to information processing. This dual engagement enhances learning and retention.

2. **Association and Connection**

- The brain processes information through associations. When new information is linked to existing knowledge, it is more easily remembered and understood. Mind mapping mimics this natural process by creating visual connections between concepts. Each branch and sub-branch represent a different association, helping to reinforce these connections and improve recall.

3. **Visual and Spatial Processing**

    - The brain is highly adept at processing visual and spatial information. Images, colors, and spatial arrangements are more memorable than plain text because they engage the brain's visual cortex. Mind maps capitalize on this by incorporating visual elements, making information more engaging and easier to remember.

4. **Chunking Information**

    - Cognitive psychology suggests that the brain can handle information more effectively when it is broken down into manageable chunks. Mind mapping naturally segments information into small, interconnected units, making complex topics more digestible and less overwhelming.

5. **Working Memory**

    o Working memory is responsible for temporarily holding and manipulating information. It plays a crucial role in tasks that require focus, organization, and problem-solving. Mind mapping reduces cognitive load by organizing information visually, which helps free up working memory and improve concentration and productivity.

How It Engages the ADHD Brain

Mind mapping is particularly effective for individuals with ADHD because it aligns with their cognitive strengths and addresses common challenges. Here's how mind mapping engages the ADHD brain:

1. **Visual Stimulation**

    o The ADHD brain often craves visual and sensory stimulation. Mind maps provide a rich visual experience through the use of colors, images, and spatial arrangements.

This visual stimulation helps maintain interest and engagement, making it easier to focus on the task at hand.

2. **Non-linear Thinking**

    o People with ADHD tend to think in a non-linear, associative manner. Traditional linear note-taking methods can feel restrictive and counterproductive. Mind mapping embraces this non-linear thinking by allowing ideas to flow freely and organically. This flexibility helps individuals with ADHD organize their thoughts in a way that makes sense to them.

3. **Active Engagement**

    o Creating a mind map is an active process that requires participation and creativity. This active engagement helps improve focus and concentration, which are often areas of difficulty for those with ADHD. The process of drawing branches, adding colors, and incorporating images keeps the mind engaged and reduces distractions.

4. **Breaking Down Tasks**
    o One of the common challenges for individuals with ADHD is breaking down large tasks into smaller, manageable steps. Mind mapping naturally segments information into smaller units, making it easier to tackle complex tasks and projects. This structured approach can reduce feelings of overwhelm and increase productivity.

5. **Enhancing Memory and Recall**
    o ADHD often comes with challenges related to memory and recall. The visual and associative nature of mind maps helps reinforce connections between ideas, improving both short-term and long-term memory. The use of keywords, images, and colors creates strong mental cues that aid in recalling information.

6. **Reducing Overwhelm**
    o The ADHD brain can easily become overwhelmed by too much information or cluttered environments. Mind maps provide a clear and organized way to

visualize information, reducing mental clutter. By presenting information in a concise and visually appealing manner, mind maps help create a sense of order and control.

7. **Stimulating Creativity**

    o Individuals with ADHD often possess high levels of creativity and out-of-the-box thinking. Mind mapping taps into this creativity by allowing for free-form expression and exploration of ideas. This creative outlet can be both motivating and therapeutic, providing a positive way to channel energy and ideas.

8. **Personalization**

    o Mind maps can be tailored to individual preferences and needs. Whether you prefer digital tools or pen and paper, you can customize your mind maps with colors, images, and layouts that resonate with you. This personalization makes mind mapping a flexible and adaptable tool that can evolve with your changing needs.

Chapter 3

Tools and Techniques

Materials Needed for Mind Mapping

Getting started with mind mapping requires minimal materials, and you can choose between traditional and digital tools based on your preference. Here's a list of essentials:

1. **Paper**:

    - **Blank Paper**: Blank sheets provide the flexibility to expand your mind map without constraints.
    - **Notebook**: A notebook dedicated to mind mapping can help you keep your ideas organized in one place.

2. **Writing Instruments**:

    - **Pens and Pencils**: Use a variety of pens and pencils for writing and drawing. Mechanical pencils are great for finer details.
    - **Colored Markers and Highlighters**: Colors can help differentiate between

branches and highlight important points, making your mind map more visually engaging and easier to understand.

3. **Extras**:

    - **Sticky Notes**: Useful for adding ideas that can be moved around as your mind map evolves.
    - **Stencils and Rulers**: While not necessary, these can help create cleaner, more structured maps if you prefer a more polished look.

Various Mind Mapping Tools and Apps

With the advancement of technology, numerous digital tools and apps are available that can enhance the mind mapping experience. Here's an overview of some popular options:

1. **MindMeister**

    - **Overview**: MindMeister is an online mind mapping tool that allows you to create, share, and collaborate on mind maps. It offers a user-friendly interface with a variety of templates and customization options.

- **Key Features**: Real-time collaboration, integration with other tools like Google Drive and Slack, and a library of pre-made templates.
- **Best For**: Collaborative projects, business planning, and educational purposes.

2. **XMind**

    - **Overview**: XMind is a versatile mind mapping software available for both desktop and mobile devices. It offers a range of features for creating detailed and visually appealing mind maps.
    - **Key Features**: Gantt charts for project planning, brainstorming modes, and various export options (e.g., PDF, Word, PowerPoint).
    - **Best For**: Comprehensive project management, individual planning, and professional presentations.

3. **SimpleMind**

    - **Overview**: SimpleMind is an intuitive mind mapping tool available on multiple platforms, including Windows, macOS, iOS, and Android. It focuses on simplicity and ease of use.

- **Key Features**: Cross-platform synchronization, various layout options, and the ability to add media (e.g., images, videos).
- **Best For**: Personal organization, brainstorming sessions, and academic note-taking.

4. **Coggle**

    - **Overview**: Coggle is an online mind mapping tool that emphasizes collaboration and simplicity. It's web-based, making it accessible from any device with an internet connection.
    - **Key Features**: Real-time collaboration, version history tracking, and easy sharing via links.
    - **Best For**: Team projects, quick brainstorming, and visualizing complex information.

5. **iMindMap (now Ayoa)**

    - **Overview**: Developed by Tony Buzan, iMindMap (now part of Ayoa) offers a comprehensive set of tools for mind mapping and task management. It

combines visual mapping with task boards and collaboration features.
- **Key Features**: 3D mind maps, radial maps, built-in task management, and integration with other productivity tools.
- **Best For**: Creative professionals, teams working on complex projects, and individuals who prefer a visual approach to task management.

6. **MindMup**

    - **Overview**: MindMup is a free, online mind mapping tool that integrates seamlessly with Google Drive. It offers a straightforward interface with essential mind mapping features.
    - **Key Features**: Google Drive integration, ability to publish maps online, and various export options.
    - **Best For**: Quick mind maps, educational purposes, and those who prefer cloud-based solutions.

7. **FreeMind**

    - **Overview**: FreeMind is an open-source mind mapping tool that offers a robust set of features for creating detailed mind

maps. It's available for Windows, macOS, and Linux.
- **Key Features**: Extensive formatting options, hyperlinks, and the ability to export in multiple formats.
- **Best For**: Users who need a powerful, free tool with extensive customization options.

How to Choose the Right Tool

Choosing the right mind mapping tool depends on your specific needs and preferences. Here are some factors to consider:

1. **Purpose**: Determine the primary purpose of your mind maps. Are they for personal use, professional projects, or collaborative efforts? Different tools cater to different needs.

2. **Ease of Use**: Consider your comfort level with technology. Some tools offer a simple, intuitive interface, while others provide more advanced features that might require a learning curve.

3. **Collaboration**: If you plan to collaborate with others, look for tools that offer real-time collaboration features and easy sharing options.

4. **Customization**: Evaluate the level of customization you need. Some tools provide extensive options for colors, layouts, and media, while others focus on simplicity.

5. **Platform Compatibility**: Ensure the tool is compatible with your devices and operating systems. Cross-platform tools can be beneficial if you need to access your mind maps on different devices.

6. **Cost**: While some tools are free, others may require a subscription or one-time purchase. Consider your budget and the value the tool provides.

By selecting the right materials and tools, you can create effective and visually engaging mind maps that enhance your productivity and creativity. Whether you prefer the tactile experience of pen and paper or the flexibility of digital tools, mind mapping can be a powerful addition to your ADHD management toolkit. In the next chapter, we will dive into the step-by-step process of creating your first mind map, providing practical tips and examples to help you get started.

Part 2

Applying Mind Mapping in Everyday Life

Chapter 4

Personal Life

Mind mapping can be an invaluable tool for managing various aspects of your personal life. From daily routines to meal planning and personal goal setting, mind maps can help you stay organized, focused, and productive. In this chapter, we will explore how to use mind mapping to streamline your daily activities and achieve your personal goals.

Managing Daily Routines and Chores

Daily routines and chores can be overwhelming, especially for individuals with ADHD who may struggle with organization and time management. Mind mapping can help you visualize and structure your daily tasks, making them more manageable and less daunting.

1. **Creating a Daily Routine Map**
    - Start with a central node labeled "Daily Routine."
    - Branch out into different categories such as "Morning Routine," "Afternoon Tasks," "Evening Routine," and "Nighttime Wind-Down."

- Under each category, list specific tasks or activities. For example, under "Morning Routine," you might include "Wake up," "Exercise," "Shower," "Breakfast," and "Plan the Day."
- Use colors and symbols to differentiate between tasks and highlight priorities.

2. **Visualizing Weekly Chores**

    - Create a separate mind map for weekly chores.
    - Begin with a central node labeled "Weekly Chores."
    - Branch out into days of the week, e.g., "Monday," "Tuesday," etc.
    - Under each day, list the chores that need to be completed, such as "Laundry," "Grocery Shopping," "Vacuuming," and "Trash Disposal."
    - Assign specific colors to each day or type of chore to make the map more visually appealing and easier to follow.

3. **Incorporating Time Estimates**

    - Add estimated time durations to each task or chore to help with time management.

- This can be done by including small notes or icons next to each task indicating how long it will take.
- This approach helps in planning your day more effectively and prevents time from slipping away on less important activities.

Meal Planning and Grocery Shopping

Meal planning and grocery shopping can become much more organized and efficient with the help of mind mapping. Here's how you can use mind maps to streamline these processes:

1. **Meal Planning Mind Map**

    - Start with a central node labeled "Meal Planning."
    - Branch out into different meal categories such as "Breakfast," "Lunch," "Dinner," and "Snacks."
    - Under each category, list specific meals or recipes you plan to prepare for the week.
    - You can further branch out from each meal with ingredients needed, cooking instructions, and any special notes (e.g., dietary restrictions or preferences).

2. **Grocery Shopping List**

    - Create a mind map for your grocery shopping list.
    - Begin with a central node labeled "Grocery Shopping."
    - Branch out into different sections of the grocery store, such as "Produce," "Dairy," "Meat," "Pantry Items," and "Household Supplies."
    - Under each section, list the items you need to purchase.
    - This method helps you visualize your shopping list in a structured way, making it easier to navigate the store and avoid forgetting items.

3. **Integrating Meal Plans and Shopping Lists**

    - Combine your meal planning mind map with your grocery shopping list.
    - Start with a central node labeled "Weekly Meals and Groceries."
    - Branch out into days of the week or meal categories.
    - Under each day or category, list the meals you plan to prepare and the corresponding ingredients.

- From the ingredients, create branches that lead to your grocery list sections.
- This integrated approach ensures that you have all the necessary ingredients for your meals and streamlines your shopping experience.

Personal Goal Setting and Tracking

Setting and tracking personal goals can be challenging, but mind mapping can provide a clear and motivating way to visualize your aspirations and progress.

1. **Goal Setting Mind Map**
    - Start with a central node labeled "Personal Goals."
    - Branch out into different areas of your life, such as "Health," "Career," "Education," "Hobbies," and "Relationships."
    - Under each area, list specific goals you want to achieve. For example, under "Health," you might include "Exercise 3 times a week," "Eat more vegetables," and "Meditate daily."
    - Use colors and images to represent each goal, making the map visually engaging and inspiring.

2. **Breaking Down Goals**

    o For each goal, create sub-branches that break down the steps needed to achieve it.
    o For example, under "Exercise 3 times a week," you might include sub-steps like "Join a gym," "Create a workout schedule," and "Track progress."
    o This approach helps you see the actionable steps required to reach your goals and makes them feel more attainable.

3. **Tracking Progress**

    o Create a mind map to track your progress on each goal.
    o Start with a central node labeled "Goal Tracking."
    o Branch out into each goal you've set, and under each goal, list the milestones or checkpoints you need to reach.
    o Use symbols or colors to indicate your progress, such as green for completed tasks, yellow for in-progress tasks, and red for tasks that need attention.
    o Regularly update your mind map to reflect your progress and adjust your plans as needed.

4. **Review and Reflect**

    o Periodically review your goal-setting mind map to reflect on your achievements and areas for improvement.
    o Use a central node labeled "Reflection" with branches for "Achievements," "Challenges," and "Next Steps."
    o Under "Achievements," list the goals you've accomplished and celebrate your successes.
    o Under "Challenges," note any obstacles you've encountered and consider ways to overcome them.
    o Under "Next Steps," outline your plans for continuing your progress and setting new goals.

By incorporating mind mapping into your personal life, you can create a visual and structured approach to managing daily routines, meal planning, and goal setting. This method not only helps you stay organized and focused but also leverages your creative strengths, making your personal journey more enjoyable and fulfilling.

Chapter 5

Professional Life

Mind mapping is a versatile tool that can significantly enhance your professional life by helping you organize tasks, boost creativity, and improve time management. In this chapter, we will explore how to use mind mapping in the workplace to stay productive, innovative, and efficient.

Organizing Tasks and Projects at Work

In a professional setting, staying organized is key to managing your workload effectively. Mind mapping can help you break down complex projects into manageable tasks and keep track of your progress.

1. **Task Management Mind Map**
    - Start with a central node labeled "Work Tasks" or "Project Name."
    - Branch out into different categories of tasks, such as "Immediate Tasks," "Upcoming Deadlines," "Ongoing Projects," and "Long-term Goals."
    - Under each category, list specific tasks that need to be completed. For example,

under "Immediate Tasks," you might include "Send email updates," "Prepare meeting agenda," and "Submit report."
- Use colors to differentiate between task categories and priority levels.

2. **Project Planning**

    - Create a separate mind map for each major project you are working on.
    - Start with a central node labeled with the project name.
    - Branch out into key components of the project, such as "Research," "Development," "Testing," "Marketing," and "Launch."
    - Under each component, list the tasks and milestones required to complete that phase of the project.
    - Include deadlines and responsible team members for each task to keep everyone accountable and on track.

3. **Progress Tracking**

    - Use mind maps to track the progress of your tasks and projects.
    - Start with a central node labeled "Progress Tracker."

- Branch out into each project or task category.
- Under each branch, list the tasks and their current status (e.g., not started, in progress, completed).
- Update the mind map regularly to reflect your progress and make adjustments as needed.

Enhancing Creativity and Brainstorming

Creativity and innovation are crucial in many professional fields. Mind mapping can facilitate brainstorming sessions and help you generate and organize ideas effectively.

1. **Brainstorming Sessions**
    - Start with a central node labeled "Brainstorming Session" or the specific topic you are brainstorming about.
    - Branch out into different categories related to the topic, such as "Ideas," "Challenges," "Solutions," and "Resources."
    - Under each category, add sub-branches for specific ideas, challenges, or solutions. For example, under "Ideas,"

you might list different strategies or concepts.
- Encourage free-flowing thought by allowing participants to add branches and sub-branches without constraints.

2. **Idea Generation**

    - Use mind maps to explore and expand on individual ideas.
    - Start with a central node labeled with the core idea.
    - Branch out into related sub-ideas, questions, and possible actions.
    - Under each sub-idea, list further details, potential outcomes, and any additional thoughts.
    - This method helps you explore the full scope of an idea and uncover new angles and opportunities.

3. **Collaborative Mind Mapping**

    - Leverage mind mapping tools that allow real-time collaboration for team brainstorming sessions.
    - Start with a shared central node labeled with the brainstorming topic.

- Invite team members to add branches and sub-branches with their ideas and input.
- Use colors and symbols to represent different contributors and categorize ideas.
- This collaborative approach ensures that all perspectives are considered and encourages team engagement.

Time Management and Prioritization

Effective time management and prioritization are essential for professional success. Mind mapping can help you allocate your time wisely and prioritize tasks efficiently.

1. **Daily and Weekly Schedules**

    - Create a mind map for your daily or weekly schedule.
    - Start with a central node labeled "Daily Schedule" or "Weekly Schedule."
    - Branch out into days of the week or specific time blocks (e.g., "Morning," "Afternoon," "Evening").
    - Under each branch, list the tasks and activities planned for that period. Include deadlines, meetings, and breaks.

- Use colors to highlight urgent tasks and priorities.

2. **Priority Mapping**

    - Use mind maps to prioritize your tasks and responsibilities.
    - Start with a central node labeled "Priorities."
    - Branch out into categories such as "High Priority," "Medium Priority," and "Low Priority."
    - Under each category, list the tasks that fall into that priority level.
    - Assign deadlines and estimated completion times to each task to help with time management.

3. **Time Blocking**

    - Create a mind map to visualize your time blocks for different tasks and activities.
    - Start with a central node labeled "Time Blocking."
    - Branch out into different categories such as "Work," "Meetings," "Breaks," and "Personal Time."

- Under each category, list the tasks and activities you plan to complete within specific time blocks.
- This method helps you allocate dedicated time for focused work, minimizing distractions and improving productivity.

4. **Project Timeline Mapping**

    - Use mind maps to create project timelines and milestones.
    - Start with a central node labeled "Project Timeline."
    - Branch out into different phases of the project, such as "Planning," "Execution," "Review," and "Completion."
    - Under each phase, list the key tasks, deadlines, and milestones.
    - Include dependencies and critical paths to ensure that you stay on track and meet project deadlines.

By incorporating mind mapping into your professional life, you can organize tasks and projects more effectively, enhance creativity, and improve time management. This structured yet flexible approach allows you to visualize your work, prioritize tasks, and stay focused on your goals.

Chapter 6

Academic Pursuits

Mind mapping can be a powerful tool for students and lifelong learners, enhancing note-taking, studying, essay writing, and exam preparation. In this chapter, we will explore how to utilize mind mapping to excel in your academic pursuits.

Note-Taking and Studying Techniques

Effective note-taking and studying are crucial for academic success. Mind mapping can transform the way you capture and review information.

1. **Mind Mapping for Note-Taking**
    - **Creating Notes**:
        - Start with a central node labeled with the topic or lecture title.
        - Branch out into main ideas or sections covered in the class or reading material.
        - Under each branch, add sub-branches for specific details, examples, and key points.

- Use colors, symbols, and images to highlight important information and make the map more visually engaging.
    - **Reviewing Notes**:
        - Use your mind maps to review and reinforce your understanding of the material.
        - Regularly revisit your maps, adding new information or clarifying points as needed.
        - Summarize key concepts in separate branches to consolidate your knowledge.

2. **Studying with Mind Maps**

    - **Organizing Study Sessions**:
        - Create a mind map to organize your study sessions.
        - Start with a central node labeled "Study Plan."
        - Branch out into different subjects or topics you need to study.
        - Under each branch, list specific study activities, such as reading chapters, solving problems, or watching lectures.

- Assign time slots and deadlines to each activity to ensure balanced and effective study sessions.
  - **Visualizing Connections**:
    - Use mind maps to visualize connections between concepts.
    - Start with a central node labeled with a broad topic or theme.
    - Branch out into related subtopics, theories, or principles.
    - Show how different concepts interrelate, which can enhance your understanding and retention of the material.

Planning and Writing Essays or Reports

Mind mapping can streamline the process of planning, organizing, and writing essays or reports, making it easier to produce well-structured and coherent work.

1. **Planning Your Essay or Report**
   - **Brainstorming Ideas**:
     - Start with a central node labeled with your essay or report topic.
     - Branch out into different ideas, arguments, or themes you want to explore.

- Under each idea, add sub-branches for supporting points, evidence, and examples.
- This brainstorming process helps you generate a wide range of ideas and choose the most compelling ones for your work.
  - **Organizing Structure**:
    - Create a mind map to outline the structure of your essay or report.
    - Start with a central node labeled "Outline."
    - Branch out into main sections such as "Introduction," "Body," and "Conclusion."
    - Under each section, list the main points you plan to cover and the order in which they will appear.
    - This visual outline helps you maintain a logical flow and ensures that all key points are addressed.

2. **Writing the Essay or Report**

   - **Developing Sections**:
     - Use your outline mind map as a guide to develop each section of your essay or report.

- Start with the introduction, expanding on the points listed in your mind map.
- Move on to the body, using each branch and sub-branch to structure your paragraphs and support your arguments.
- Conclude by summarizing the main points and reinforcing your thesis or purpose.

○ **Revising and Editing**:
- Create a mind map to plan your revision and editing process.
- Start with a central node labeled "Revision Plan."
- Branch out into different aspects of your work, such as "Content," "Structure," "Grammar," and "Style."
- Under each branch, list specific tasks for revising and improving your work, such as checking for clarity, reorganizing sections, and correcting errors.
- This structured approach ensures a thorough and efficient revision process.

Preparing for Exams

Exam preparation can be stressful, but mind mapping can help you organize your study materials, review key concepts, and retain information more effectively.

1. **Creating Study Guides**
    - **Summarizing Content**:
        - Start with a central node labeled with the exam subject or topic.
        - Branch out into major themes or units covered in the course.
        - Under each theme, add sub-branches for key concepts, definitions, formulas, and important details.
        - Use colors and images to highlight critical information and make the study guide more memorable.
    - **Mapping Previous Exams**:
        - Create a mind map based on previous exam questions or topics.
        - Start with a central node labeled "Previous Exams."
        - Branch out into different sections, each representing a past exam or set of questions.

- Under each section, list the questions or topics covered and add branches for the answers or relevant information.
- This practice helps you identify patterns and focus on areas that are likely to be tested.

2. **Reviewing and Retaining Information**

    o **Active Recall Practice**:
       - Use mind maps to practice active recall, a proven technique for enhancing memory.
       - Start with a central node labeled "Review."
       - Branch out into key topics or questions you need to recall.
       - Cover the sub-branches and try to recall the information from memory before checking your mind map for accuracy.
       - This technique strengthens your recall ability and reinforces your understanding of the material.
    o **Spaced Repetition**:
       - Create a mind map to plan your spaced repetition schedule.

- Start with a central node labeled "Spaced Repetition."
- Branch out into different study sessions, each representing a review interval (e.g., one day, one week, one month).
- Under each session, list the topics or concepts you need to review.
- Spaced repetition helps you reinforce knowledge at optimal intervals, improving long-term retention.

3. **Practice Tests and Simulations**

   - **Simulating Exam Conditions**:
     - Use mind maps to create practice tests and simulate exam conditions.
     - Start with a central node labeled "Practice Test."
     - Branch out into different sections, each representing a part of the exam (e.g., multiple choice, essays, problem-solving).
     - Under each section, list practice questions or problems.
     - Take the practice test under timed conditions to get used to the exam

format and improve your time management skills.
- **Analyzing Performance**:
  - Create a mind map to analyze your performance on practice tests.
  - Start with a central node labeled "Test Analysis."
  - Branch out into different aspects of your performance, such as "Strengths," "Weaknesses," "Common Mistakes," and "Areas for Improvement."
  - Under each branch, list specific observations and actions you can take to improve your performance.
  - This analysis helps you identify gaps in your knowledge and develop strategies to address them.

By incorporating mind mapping into your academic pursuits, you can enhance your note-taking, studying, essay writing, and exam preparation techniques. This visual and structured approach makes learning more engaging and effective, helping you achieve academic success. In the next part of the book, we will explore how mind mapping can be applied to personal development, offering practical strategies to help you achieve a balanced and fulfilling life.

Part 3

Personal Development Through Mind Mapping

Chapter 7

Self-Care and Mindfulness

Self-care and mindfulness are essential components of maintaining overall well-being, especially for women with ADHD. Mind mapping can be a powerful tool to plan and track self-care routines and monitor your mood and emotional triggers. In this chapter, we will explore how to incorporate mind mapping into your self-care and mindfulness practices.

Using Mind Maps to Plan Self-Care Routines

Creating a structured self-care routine can help you prioritize your well-being and ensure you take time to nurture yourself amidst daily responsibilities.

1. **Designing Your Self-Care Routine**

    - **Creating a Self-Care Map**:
        - Start with a central node labeled "Self-Care Routine."
        - Branch out into different categories of self-care, such as "Physical Health," "Mental Health," "Emotional Well-being,"

"Social Connections," and "Leisure Activities."
- Under each category, list specific self-care activities. For example, under "Physical Health," you might include "Exercise," "Healthy Eating," "Sleep," and "Hydration."
- Use colors and symbols to differentiate between categories and highlight activities that are particularly important to you.

o **Daily and Weekly Planning**:
- Create separate branches for daily, weekly, and monthly self-care activities.
- Under "Daily," list activities such as "Morning Stretch," "Meditation," "Healthy Breakfast," and "Journaling."
- Under "Weekly," include activities like "Yoga Class," "Therapy Session," "Nature Walk," and "Catch-up with Friends."
- Under "Monthly," you might list activities like "Spa Day," "Book Club," and "Personal Reflection."

2. **Setting Self-Care Goals**

   o **Short-term and Long-term Goals**:
      - Start with a central node labeled "Self-Care Goals."
      - Branch out into "Short-term Goals" and "Long-term Goals."
      - Under each branch, list specific goals. For example, a short-term goal might be "Exercise 3 times a week," while a long-term goal could be "Run a 5K."
   o **Action Steps**:
      - For each goal, create sub-branches that outline the steps needed to achieve it.
      - For example, under "Exercise 3 times a week," you might include steps like "Join a gym," "Create a workout schedule," and "Track progress."
      - This detailed approach helps you break down your goals into manageable tasks and stay motivated.

3. **Visualizing Your Self-Care Journey**
    - **Progress Tracking**:
        - Create a mind map to track your progress with self-care activities and goals.
        - Start with a central node labeled "Self-Care Progress."
        - Branch out into different time frames, such as "Daily," "Weekly," and "Monthly."
        - Under each time frame, list the activities you have completed and any observations or reflections.
        - Use symbols or colors to indicate completed activities and milestones reached.
    - **Reflection and Adjustment**:
        - Periodically review your self-care mind map to reflect on what's working and what needs adjustment.
        - Create a branch labeled "Reflection" with sub-branches for "Successes," "Challenges," and "Improvements."

- Under "Successes," list the activities and goals you've achieved.
- Under "Challenges," note any difficulties or barriers you've encountered.
- Under "Improvements," outline changes or new strategies to enhance your self-care routine.

Tracking Mood and Emotional Triggers

Understanding and managing your mood and emotional triggers is crucial for maintaining mental and emotional well-being. Mind mapping can help you track patterns and develop coping strategies.

1. **Mood Tracking**

    - **Creating a Mood Map**:
        - Start with a central node labeled "Mood Tracker."
        - Branch out into different moods or emotions you experience, such as "Happy," "Anxious," "Sad," "Excited," and "Frustrated."
        - Under each mood, list specific events, situations, or activities that typically trigger that mood.

- Use colors to represent different moods, making the map visually clear and easy to interpret.
    - **Daily Mood Log**:
        - Create a daily mood log mind map.
        - Start with a central node labeled "Daily Mood Log."
        - Branch out into days of the week.
        - Under each day, list the predominant mood(s) you experienced and any significant events or triggers.
        - This daily tracking helps you identify patterns and understand how different factors influence your mood.

2. **Identifying Emotional Triggers**
    - **Mapping Triggers**:
        - Create a mind map focused on emotional triggers.
        - Start with a central node labeled "Emotional Triggers."
        - Branch out into different categories of triggers, such as "Work Stress," "Relationship Issues," "Health Concerns,"

"Financial Worries," and "Environmental Factors."
- Under each category, list specific triggers. For example, under "Work Stress," you might include "Deadlines," "High Workload," and "Conflicts with Colleagues."
- **Developing Coping Strategies**:
  - For each trigger, create sub-branches that outline coping strategies.
  - For example, under "Deadlines," you might list strategies like "Prioritize Tasks," "Break Work into Smaller Steps," and "Take Short Breaks."
  - This approach helps you prepare for and manage emotional triggers effectively.

3. **Reflecting on Emotional Patterns**

   - **Creating an Emotion Reflection Map**:
     - Start with a central node labeled "Emotional Reflection."
     - Branch out into different time frames, such as "Daily," "Weekly," and "Monthly."

- Under each time frame, list the predominant emotions you experienced and any significant insights or reflections.
    - Use symbols or colors to highlight recurring patterns or significant emotional shifts.
  - **Identifying Trends**:
    - Create a mind map to identify trends in your emotional patterns.
    - Start with a central node labeled "Emotion Trends."
    - Branch out into different categories such as "Positive Trends" and "Negative Trends."
    - Under each category, list specific trends you've noticed. For example, under "Positive Trends," you might include "Increased Happiness with Regular Exercise."
    - This analysis helps you understand how different factors influence your emotions and adjust your self-care strategies accordingly.

By incorporating mind mapping into your self-care and mindfulness practices, you can create structured routines, track your mood and emotional triggers, and develop effective coping strategies. This visual and organized approach helps you prioritize your well-being and achieve a balanced, fulfilling life.

Chapter 8

Stress Management

Managing stress is vital for maintaining mental and physical health, particularly for women with ADHD. Mind mapping can be a valuable tool for identifying stressors, exploring coping mechanisms, and organizing relaxation techniques. This chapter will guide you on how to use mind mapping to effectively manage stress.

Identifying Stressors and Coping Mechanisms

Understanding the sources of your stress and developing strategies to manage them can significantly reduce their impact on your life.

1. **Identifying Stressors**

    - **Creating a Stressor Map**:
        - Start with a central node labeled "Stressors."
        - Branch out into different categories of stressors, such as "Work," "Relationships," "Health," "Finances," and "Daily Life."

- Under each category, list specific stressors. For example, under "Work," you might include "Deadlines," "Overtime," "Workload," and "Conflict with Colleagues."
            - Use colors to differentiate between categories and highlight particularly severe or frequent stressors.
        o **Tracking Stressors Over Time**:
            - Create a mind map to track stressors over time.
            - Start with a central node labeled "Stress Tracker."
            - Branch out into different time frames, such as "Daily," "Weekly," and "Monthly."
            - Under each time frame, list the stressors you encountered and their impact on your mood and well-being.
            - This tracking helps you identify patterns and understand how different factors influence your stress levels.

2. **Exploring Coping Mechanisms**

- **Mapping Coping Strategies**:
    - Start with a central node labeled "Coping Mechanisms."
    - Branch out into different categories of coping strategies, such as "Physical Activities," "Mental Techniques," "Emotional Support," and "Practical Solutions."
    - Under each category, list specific strategies. For example, under "Physical Activities," you might include "Exercise," "Yoga," "Walking," and "Deep Breathing."
    - Use colors and symbols to represent different types of coping mechanisms and their effectiveness.
- **Personalizing Coping Strategies**:
    - Create a mind map to personalize your coping strategies.
    - Start with a central node labeled "My Coping Strategies."
    - Branch out into different stressors or categories of stress.
    - Under each branch, list the coping mechanisms you have found

effective for managing that particular stressor.
- This personalized approach helps you develop a tailored stress management plan that works best for you.

Creating a Mind Map for Relaxation Techniques

Relaxation techniques are essential for reducing stress and promoting overall well-being. Mind mapping can help you explore and organize various relaxation methods.

1. **Exploring Relaxation Techniques**

    o **Creating a Relaxation Map**:
       - Start with a central node labeled "Relaxation Techniques."
       - Branch out into different categories of relaxation methods, such as "Physical Relaxation," "Mental Relaxation," "Sensory Relaxation," and "Creative Relaxation."
       - Under each category, list specific techniques. For example, under

"Physical Relaxation," you might include "Progressive Muscle Relaxation," "Stretching," "Massage," and "Warm Bath."
- Use colors and symbols to differentiate between categories and highlight techniques that you find particularly soothing.
  - **Detailing Techniques**:
    - For each relaxation technique, create sub-branches that outline the steps or components of the technique.
    - For example, under "Progressive Muscle Relaxation," you might list steps such as "Find a Quiet Space," "Sit or Lie Down Comfortably," "Tense Muscle Groups," and "Relax Muscle Groups."
    - This detailed approach helps you understand and practice each technique effectively.

2. **Planning Relaxation Sessions**

    - **Scheduling Relaxation Time**:
      - Create a mind map to plan and schedule relaxation sessions.

- Start with a central node labeled "Relaxation Schedule."
- Branch out into different time frames, such as "Daily," "Weekly," and "Monthly."
- Under each time frame, list the relaxation techniques you plan to practice and the specific times you will dedicate to them.
- This planning ensures that you regularly take time to relax and recharge.

○ **Combining Techniques**:
- Use a mind map to combine different relaxation techniques into a comprehensive relaxation routine.
- Start with a central node labeled "Relaxation Routine."
- Branch out into different time blocks, such as "Morning," "Afternoon," and "Evening."
- Under each time block, list the relaxation techniques you plan to practice.
- For example, your "Morning" routine might include "Meditation" and "Stretching,"

while your "Evening" routine might include "Warm Bath" and "Reading."
- This comprehensive approach helps you integrate relaxation into your daily life.

3. **Reflecting on Relaxation Techniques**
    - **Creating a Reflection Map**:
        - Start with a central node labeled "Relaxation Reflection."
        - Branch out into different time frames, such as "Daily," "Weekly," and "Monthly."
        - Under each time frame, list the relaxation techniques you practiced and their impact on your stress levels and well-being.
        - Use symbols or colors to indicate the effectiveness of each technique and any adjustments you plan to make.
    - **Identifying Trends and Adjustments**:
        - Create a mind map to identify trends and make adjustments to your relaxation techniques.
        - Start with a central node labeled "Relaxation Trends."

- Branch out into different categories, such as "Most Effective Techniques," "Less Effective Techniques," and "New Techniques to Try."
- Under each category, list specific observations and adjustments. For example, under "Most Effective Techniques," you might include "Deep Breathing before Sleep."
- This analysis helps you refine your relaxation practices and discover what works best for you.

By incorporating mind mapping into your stress management practices, you can identify stressors, develop effective coping mechanisms, and explore various relaxation techniques. This structured and visual approach helps you manage stress more effectively, promoting a balanced and healthy lifestyle.

Chapter 9

Building Healthy Relationships

Healthy relationships are vital for emotional well-being and overall happiness, especially for women with ADHD who may face unique challenges in communication and relationship dynamics. Mind mapping can be a powerful tool to improve communication strategies and understand relationship dynamics. This chapter will guide you on how to use mind mapping to foster healthy relationships.

Mapping Out Communication Strategies

Effective communication is the foundation of any healthy relationship. Mind mapping can help you develop and visualize strategies to enhance your communication skills.

1. **Identifying Communication Styles**

    - **Creating a Communication Style Map**:
        - Start with a central node labeled "Communication Styles."
        - Branch out into different communication styles, such as "Assertive," "Passive,"

"Aggressive," and "Passive-Aggressive."
- Under each style, list characteristics and examples. For example, under "Assertive," you might include "Expresses needs clearly," "Respects others," and "Maintains eye contact."
- Use colors and symbols to differentiate between styles and highlight the one you aim to adopt.

o **Self-Assessment**:
- Create a mind map to assess your current communication style.
- Start with a central node labeled "My Communication Style."
- Branch out into different situations, such as "At Work," "With Family," "With Friends," and "In Conflict."
- Under each situation, list your typical communication behaviors and identify any patterns or areas for improvement.

2. **Developing Effective Communication Techniques**

- **Mapping Communication Techniques**:
  - Start with a central node labeled "Communication Techniques."
  - Branch out into different techniques, such as "Active Listening," "Clear Expression," "Non-Verbal Communication," and "Feedback."
  - Under each technique, list specific strategies. For example, under "Active Listening," you might include "Maintain eye contact," "Nod to show understanding," and "Paraphrase to confirm understanding."
  - Use colors and symbols to emphasize key strategies and techniques.
- **Creating Communication Plans**:
  - Use a mind map to develop communication plans for specific situations.
  - Start with a central node labeled "Communication Plan."
  - Branch out into different scenarios, such as "Discussing Needs," "Resolving Conflicts," and "Giving Feedback."

- Under each scenario, list the steps and techniques you will use to communicate effectively.
- For example, under "Resolving Conflicts," you might include steps like "Stay calm," "Listen actively," "Express feelings clearly," and "Seek a mutually beneficial solution."

3. **Improving Non-Verbal Communication**

    o **Mapping Non-Verbal Cues**:
    - Create a mind map to explore non-verbal communication cues.
    - Start with a central node labeled "Non-Verbal Communication."
    - Branch out into different types of non-verbal cues, such as "Body Language," "Facial Expressions," "Gestures," and "Tone of Voice."
    - Under each type, list specific cues and their meanings. For example, under "Body Language," you might include "Crossed arms (defensive)," "Open posture (receptive)," and "Leaning forward (interest)."

- Use images or icons to visually represent each cue.
- **Practicing Non-Verbal Communication**:
  - Create a mind map to practice and improve your non-verbal communication skills.
  - Start with a central node labeled "Non-Verbal Practice."
  - Branch out into different areas, such as "Eye Contact," "Posture," "Gestures," and "Facial Expressions."
  - Under each area, list specific exercises or practices. For example, under "Eye Contact," you might include "Maintain eye contact for 5 seconds," "Practice with a mirror," and "Observe others."
  - This structured approach helps you enhance your non-verbal communication and make your interactions more effective.

Understanding Relationship Dynamics

Understanding the dynamics of your relationships can help you navigate them more effectively and foster healthier connections.

1. **Mapping Relationship Dynamics**
    - **Creating a Relationship Map**:
        - Start with a central node labeled "Relationship Dynamics."
        - Branch out into different types of relationships, such as "Family," "Friends," "Romantic Partners," and "Colleagues."
        - Under each type, list the key dynamics and interactions. For example, under "Family," you might include "Parental expectations," "Sibling rivalry," and "Communication patterns."
        - Use colors and symbols to represent positive and negative dynamics.
    - **Analyzing Relationship Patterns**:
        - Create a mind map to analyze patterns in your relationships.

- Start with a central node labeled "Relationship Patterns."
- Branch out into different factors, such as "Communication," "Conflict," "Support," and "Boundaries."
- Under each factor, list specific patterns you have observed in different relationships.
- For example, under "Conflict," you might note patterns like "Avoidance in romantic relationships" or "Frequent arguments with siblings."
- This analysis helps you identify areas for improvement and understand the underlying dynamics of your relationships.

2. **Setting Boundaries**

   o **Mapping Boundaries**:
     - Start with a central node labeled "Setting Boundaries."
     - Branch out into different areas where you need to set boundaries, such as "Emotional," "Physical," "Time," and "Personal Space."

- Under each area, list specific boundaries. For example, under "Emotional," you might include "Express feelings openly," "Limit negative interactions," and "Seek mutual respect."
- Use colors and symbols to represent different types of boundaries and their importance.

○ **Communicating Boundaries**:
- Create a mind map to plan how to communicate your boundaries.
- Start with a central node labeled "Communicating Boundaries."
- Branch out into different scenarios, such as "With Family," "With Friends," "At Work," and "In Romantic Relationships."
- Under each scenario, list the steps and strategies you will use to communicate your boundaries clearly and assertively.
- For example, under "At Work," you might include steps like "Schedule a meeting," "Explain the boundary," "Provide reasons," and "Seek agreement."

- This structured approach helps you effectively communicate your boundaries and ensure they are respected.

3. **Enhancing Relationship Quality**
    - **Mapping Relationship Goals**:
        - Start with a central node labeled "Relationship Goals."
        - Branch out into different types of relationships, such as "Family," "Friends," "Romantic Partners," and "Colleagues."
        - Under each type, list specific goals you want to achieve. For example, under "Friends," you might include "Spend more quality time together," "Be more supportive," and "Resolve conflicts amicably."
        - Use colors and symbols to represent short-term and long-term goals.
    - **Planning Relationship Activities**:
        - Create a mind map to plan activities that enhance the quality of your relationships.

- Start with a central node labeled "Relationship Activities."
- Branch out into different types of activities, such as "Quality Time," "Supportive Actions," "Conflict Resolution," and "Celebrations."
- Under each type, list specific activities. For example, under "Quality Time," you might include "Weekly coffee dates," "Shared hobbies," and "Regular check-ins."
- This planning helps you prioritize and invest in activities that strengthen your relationships.

By incorporating mind mapping into your relationship-building practices, you can improve communication, understand relationship dynamics, and foster healthier connections. This structured and visual approach helps you navigate relationships more effectively, promoting emotional well-being and overall happiness.

Part 4

Real-Life Success Stories

Chapter 10

Interviews with Women Who Use Mind Mapping

In this chapter, we will explore the real-life success stories of women from various backgrounds who have harnessed the power of mind mapping to transform their lives. These interviews highlight the diverse ways in which mind mapping can impact personal, professional, and academic pursuits, offering inspiration and practical insights for your own journey.

Success Stories from Various Backgrounds

1. **Sarah: The Entrepreneur**
    - **Background**: Sarah is a successful entrepreneur who runs her own marketing agency. Diagnosed with ADHD in her late 20s, Sarah struggled with organizing her thoughts and managing her business efficiently.

- **Challenges**:
  - Difficulty prioritizing tasks
  - Overwhelm with project management
  - Communication challenges with her team

- **How Mind Mapping Helped**:
  - **Task Prioritization**: Sarah uses mind maps to break down her daily and weekly tasks. She starts with a central node for the week and branches out into client projects, internal tasks, and personal commitments. This visual organization helps her prioritize effectively.
  - **Project Management**: For each client project, Sarah creates a detailed mind map outlining the project timeline, milestones, deliverables, and team responsibilities. This structure keeps her team aligned and projects on track.
  - **Team Communication**: Sarah conducts brainstorming sessions

with her team using mind maps. This collaborative tool allows everyone to contribute ideas and visualize the project's progress, improving overall communication and collaboration.

- **Impact on Life**: Mind mapping has enabled Sarah to manage her business more effectively, reduce stress, and foster a more productive and cohesive team environment.

2. **Emily: The Graduate Student**

    - **Background**: Emily is a graduate student in psychology who was diagnosed with ADHD during her undergraduate studies. She faced challenges with staying organized, managing her coursework, and preparing for exams.

    - **Challenges**:
        - Organizing extensive research materials
        - Planning and writing thesis

- Exam preparation

  o **How Mind Mapping Helped**:
    - **Research Organization**: Emily uses mind maps to organize her research materials. She creates a central node for her thesis topic and branches out into various subtopics, listing key articles, theories, and findings under each branch. This method allows her to see connections between different pieces of information and structure her literature review effectively.
    - **Thesis Planning**: For her thesis, Emily creates a detailed mind map outlining each chapter and section. She breaks down each part into smaller tasks, such as literature review, methodology, data analysis, and discussion. This breakdown helps her manage her time and progress steadily.
    - **Exam Preparation**: Emily creates mind maps for each subject, summarizing key concepts,

theories, and important details. This visual summary helps her review efficiently and retain information better.

- **Impact on Life**: Mind mapping has helped Emily stay organized, manage her academic workload, and achieve academic success with less stress and greater confidence.

3. **Lily: The Working Mom**

    - **Background**: Lily is a working mother of two who juggles her career in finance with family responsibilities. Diagnosed with ADHD in her early 30s, Lily struggled with balancing her work and home life.

    - **Challenges**:
        - Time management between work and family
        - Planning family activities and responsibilities
        - Managing household chores

- **How Mind Mapping Helped**:
  - **Time Management**: Lily uses mind maps to plan her weekly schedule. She creates a central node for the week and branches out into work tasks, family activities, and personal time. This helps her allocate time effectively and ensures a balance between her professional and personal life.
  - **Family Planning**: For family activities and responsibilities, Lily creates a mind map that includes branches for each family member's schedule, chores, and activities. This collaborative approach helps her family stay organized and ensures everyone knows their responsibilities.
  - **Household Management**: Lily creates mind maps for household chores, breaking them down into daily, weekly, and monthly tasks. This visual organization helps her manage the household more efficiently and delegate tasks to family members.

- **Impact on Life**: Mind mapping has enabled Lily to achieve a better work-life balance, reduce overwhelm, and create a more organized and harmonious family life.

4. **Maya: The Creative Professional**

    - **Background**: Maya is a graphic designer who works freelance. Diagnosed with ADHD in her teens, Maya faced challenges with staying focused on projects, managing deadlines, and fostering creativity.

    - **Challenges**:
        - Maintaining focus on design projects
        - Meeting client deadlines
        - Stimulating creative ideas

    - **How Mind Mapping Helped**:
        - **Project Focus**: Maya uses mind maps to outline each design project. She creates a central node for the project and branches out

into client requirements, design ideas, timelines, and deliverables. This structure keeps her focused and ensures she meets client expectations.
- **Deadline Management**: For each project, Maya creates a detailed timeline mind map. She breaks down the project into phases and tasks, assigning deadlines to each. This visual plan helps her stay on track and meet deadlines consistently.
- **Fostering Creativity**: Maya uses mind maps for brainstorming design ideas. She starts with a central theme and branches out into different concepts, color schemes, and design elements. This free-flowing visualization stimulates her creativity and helps her generate unique ideas.

○ **Impact on Life**: Mind mapping has helped Maya stay focused on her projects, manage her time effectively, and enhance her creativity, leading to a successful freelance career.

How Mind Mapping Has Impacted Their Lives

The success stories of Sarah, Emily, Lily, and Maya demonstrate the transformative power of mind mapping for women with ADHD. By incorporating mind mapping into their daily routines, these women have been able to:

- **Enhance Organization**: Mind mapping provides a visual and structured way to organize tasks, projects, and responsibilities, reducing overwhelm and improving efficiency.
- **Improve Time Management**: By breaking down tasks and scheduling activities, mind mapping helps manage time more effectively and ensures a balance between different areas of life.
- **Boost Creativity**: Mind mapping stimulates creative thinking and idea generation, making it easier to brainstorm and develop innovative solutions.
- **Strengthen Communication**: Mind mapping facilitates clearer and more effective communication, whether in professional settings or personal relationships.

- **Achieve Goals**: By setting clear goals and outlining actionable steps, mind mapping helps women with ADHD stay focused and motivated, leading to the successful achievement of their aspirations.

These stories highlight that mind mapping is not just a tool for organization but a powerful strategy for personal and professional growth. In the next chapters, we will explore more real-life examples and provide practical tips on how you can apply mind mapping to various aspects of your life, empowering you on your ADHD journey.

Chapter 11

Personal Testimonies

In this chapter, we present anonymous accounts from readers who have embraced mind mapping as a tool for managing their ADHD. These personal testimonies offer practical tips, lessons learned, and advice for newcomers. Each story reflects the unique challenges and victories experienced by women with ADHD, demonstrating the diverse ways mind mapping can be integrated into daily life.

Anonymous Accounts and Tips from Readers

1. **Account 1: The Busy Professional**

    - **Challenges**: Balancing a demanding career with personal life.

    - **How Mind Mapping Helped**:
        - **Daily Task Management**: "I use a daily mind map to list my tasks. Each day, I start with a central node labeled with the date and

branch out into different categories: Work, Personal, and Errands. This structure helps me visualize my day and prioritize tasks."
- **Meeting Preparation**: "Before important meetings, I create a mind map to outline the agenda, key points, and questions I need to ask. This preparation makes me feel more confident and ensures I don't forget anything important."

- **Tips**: "Start small. Use mind mapping for daily tasks first, and once you're comfortable, expand to bigger projects. Also, keep your maps simple and uncluttered to avoid feeling overwhelmed."

2. **Account 2: The Stay-at-Home Mom**

    - **Challenges**: Managing household responsibilities and caring for children.

- **How Mind Mapping Helped**:
    - **Chore Management**: "I created a mind map for household chores, divided into daily, weekly, and monthly tasks. Each family member has their own branch with assigned tasks. This visual schedule makes it easier for everyone to understand their responsibilities."
    - **Family Activities**: "We use mind maps to plan family activities and outings. Each map includes potential activities, locations, and necessary preparations. This has made planning fun and engaging for the whole family."

- **Tips**: "Involve your family in the process. When everyone contributes to the mind map, it creates a sense of shared responsibility and makes tasks feel less burdensome."

3. **Account 3: The Student**
    - **Challenges**: Staying organized with coursework and exam preparation.

    - **How Mind Mapping Helped**:
        - **Study Plans**: "I use mind maps to create study plans for each subject. I start with the subject name in the center and branch out into topics, subtopics, and key concepts. This helps me see the big picture and ensures I cover all necessary material."
        - **Essay Writing**: "For essay assignments, I outline my thesis, main arguments, and supporting evidence using a mind map. This method keeps my writing focused and well-structured."

    - **Tips**: "Use different colors for different branches to visually separate topics. It makes your mind map more engaging and easier to navigate during study sessions."

4. **Account 4: The Artist**
    - **Challenges**: Managing creative projects and finding inspiration.

    - **How Mind Mapping Helped**:
        - **Project Planning**: "I map out each art project, starting with a central theme and branching out into materials, techniques, and deadlines. This helps me stay organized and track my progress."
        - **Idea Generation**: "When I'm looking for inspiration, I create mind maps to brainstorm themes and concepts. Each branch explores a different idea, which helps spark my creativity."

    - **Tips**: "Don't be afraid to let your mind maps be messy and colorful. The creative process can be chaotic, and mind maps should reflect that. Use them as a space to freely explore ideas."

Lessons Learned and Advice for Newcomers

1. **Embrace Flexibility**

   - **Lesson**: "Mind maps are incredibly flexible. They can be as detailed or as simple as you need them to be. Don't worry about getting it perfect; let your mind maps evolve with you."
   - **Advice**: "Start with a simple map for a single task or project. As you become more comfortable, you can add more details and complexity."

2. **Consistency is Key**

   - **Lesson**: "Consistency in using mind maps is crucial. The more you use them, the more natural and effective they become."
   - **Advice**: "Make mind mapping a daily habit. Set aside a few minutes each day to update your maps and plan your tasks."

3. **Personalize Your Mind Maps**

   - **Lesson**: "Mind maps should reflect your personal style and preferences. Customize them to suit your needs."

- **Advice**: "Use colors, symbols, and images that resonate with you. This personalization makes mind mapping more enjoyable and meaningful."

4. **Integrate Mind Maps with Other Tools**

    - **Lesson**: "Mind maps can be integrated with other organizational tools like calendars and to-do lists for enhanced effectiveness."
    - **Advice**: "Use mind maps to brainstorm and plan, then transfer actionable items to your calendar or task manager. This integration keeps you organized and on track."

5. **Use Mind Maps for Reflection**

    - **Lesson**: "Mind maps are not just for planning; they are also great for reflection and review."
    - **Advice**: "Create mind maps to reflect on completed projects or personal goals. Analyze what worked well and what could be improved. This practice helps you learn and grow."

In the next chapter, we will delve into advanced mind mapping techniques and explore how to maximize the benefits of this powerful tool in various aspects of life.

Part 5

Getting Started with Your Own Mind Mapping Journey

Chapter 12

Step-by-Step Guide to Creating Your First Mind Map

Embarking on your mind mapping journey can be an exciting and transformative experience. This chapter provides a step-by-step guide to help you create your first mind map, complete with detailed instructions, examples, and tips for overcoming initial hurdles. Whether you're new to mind mapping or looking to refine your skills, these practical steps will set you on the path to success.

Detailed instructions and examples

1. **Choose Your Topic**

   - **Start Simple**: Select a topic that is straightforward and relevant to your current needs. This could be a daily to-do list, a project plan, or brainstorming ideas for a personal goal.
   - **Example**: Let's create a mind map for planning a weekend trip.

2. **Gather Your Materials**

    - **Tools Needed**: You can create a mind map using paper and colored pens, or you can use digital tools such as mind mapping software or apps.
    - **Examples of Digital Tools**: MindMeister, XMind, MindNode, and FreeMind.

3. **Create the Central Node**

    - **Start at the Center**: In the middle of your page or digital canvas, write down the main topic. This central node is the starting point of your mind map.
    - **Example**: Write "Weekend Trip" in the center and draw a circle around it.

4. **Add Main Branches**

    - **Identify Key Categories**: Think about the main categories related to your topic. These will be the first-level branches radiating from the central node.
    - **Example**: For the "Weekend Trip," you might have branches like "Destination," "Accommodation," "Activities," and "Packing List."

5. **Expand with Sub-Branches**

    o **Break Down Categories**: For each main branch, add sub-branches to break down the category into smaller, more specific details.
    o **Example**: Under "Destination," add sub-branches like "City," "Transport," and "Travel Time." Under "Accommodation," add "Hotel Options," "Booking Details," and "Budget."

6. **Use Colors and Images**

    o **Enhance Visual Appeal**: Use different colors for each branch to make your mind map visually appealing and easier to navigate. Add images or icons to represent key points.
    o **Example**: Use blue for the "Destination" branch, green for "Accommodation," and so on. Add an image of a suitcase next to "Packing List."

7. **Review and Revise**

    o **Check for Completeness**: Review your mind map to ensure all relevant details

are included. Revise and add more branches or sub-branches if needed.
- **Example**: Make sure you've covered all aspects of your trip planning, from travel arrangements to packing essentials.

Tips for Overcoming Initial Hurdles

1. **Start Small and Simple**

    - **Advice**: Begin with a small, manageable topic to avoid feeling overwhelmed. As you become more comfortable with mind mapping, you can tackle more complex topics.
    - **Example**: Start with a daily to-do list before moving on to project planning.

2. **Practice Regularly**

    - **Advice**: Make mind mapping a regular practice. The more you use it, the more natural it will become. Set aside time each day or week to create mind maps for different purposes.
    - **Example**: Use mind mapping to plan your weekly schedule or brainstorm ideas for a new project.

3. **Experiment with Different Tools**

    - **Advice**: Try different mind mapping tools to find the one that works best for you. Experiment with both paper-based and digital options to see which you prefer.
    - **Example**: Use a notebook and colored pens for some mind maps and try digital apps like MindMeister or XMind for others.

4. **Don't Strive for Perfection**

    - **Advice**: Remember that mind maps are personal and can be as messy or as neat as you like. Focus on capturing your ideas rather than creating a perfect visual.
    - **Example**: Allow yourself to create rough drafts and refine them later if needed.

5. **Use Templates and Examples**

    - **Advice**: Look for mind map templates and examples to get inspiration and understand different ways to structure your maps. Many mind mapping tools offer pre-made templates for various purposes.

- **Example**: Use a travel planning template as a starting point for your weekend trip mind map.

6. **Incorporate Feedback**

    - **Advice**: If you're using mind maps for collaborative projects, seek feedback from others. This can provide new perspectives and help improve your mind maps.
    - **Example**: Share your project mind map with colleagues and ask for their input and suggestions.

Example: Creating a Weekend Trip Mind Map

1. **Central Node**: Write "Weekend Trip" in the center.
2. **Main Branches**:
    - **Destination**: City, Transport, Travel Time
    - **Accommodation**: Hotel Options, Booking Details, Budget
    - **Activities**: Sightseeing, Dining, Entertainment
    - **Packing List**: Clothing, Toiletries, Essentials
3. **Sub-Branches**:
    - **Destination**:

- City: Paris
- Transport: Train
- Travel Time: 3 hours
- **Accommodation**:
  - Hotel Options: Hilton, Marriott
  - Booking Details: Confirmation Number, Check-in Time
  - Budget: $300
- **Activities**:
  - Sightseeing: Eiffel Tower, Louvre Museum
  - Dining: Café de Flore, Le Jules Verne
  - Entertainment: Seine River Cruise, Moulin Rouge
- **Packing List**:
  - Clothing: Jeans, T-Shirts, Jacket
  - Toiletries: Toothbrush, Shampoo
  - Essentials: Passport, Wallet, Phone Charger

By following these steps and tips, you can create effective mind maps that help organize your thoughts, manage tasks, and achieve your goals. Mind mapping is a versatile tool that can be tailored to fit your unique needs and preferences, empowering you to harness your brain's full potential and navigate your ADHD journey with confidence.

Chapter 13

Developing a Mind Mapping Habit

Creating a habit of mind mapping can be a game-changer for women with ADHD. Establishing this practice consistently will help you manage daily tasks, reduce stress, and improve overall productivity. This chapter provides strategies for maintaining consistency and motivation, setting realistic goals, and celebrating progress.

Strategies for Consistency and Motivation

1. **Start with a Routine**

   - **Advice**: Integrate mind mapping into your daily or weekly routine. Consistency is key to developing any new habit.
   - **Example**: Set aside 10-15 minutes each morning or evening to create or update your mind maps. This could be part of your daily planning or reflection time.

2. **Use Reminders and Alarms**

- **Advice**: Use reminders or alarms to prompt you to work on your mind maps. Consistent prompts can help reinforce the habit.
- **Example**: Set a daily reminder on your phone or calendar to spend time mind mapping. Label it as "Mind Mapping Time" to create a dedicated space for this activity.

3. **Create a Dedicated Space**

    - **Advice**: Designate a specific place for mind mapping. Having a consistent location can make it easier to associate that space with the activity.
    - **Example**: Set up a cozy corner with a comfortable chair, a table, and your mind mapping materials. If you prefer digital tools, have your device ready with the mind mapping app open.

4. **Incorporate Mind Mapping into Existing Habits**

    - **Advice**: Link mind mapping with an established habit to make it easier to adopt.

- **Example**: If you have a habit of drinking coffee in the morning, pair it with a quick mind mapping session. Over time, the two activities will become naturally connected.

5. **Keep it Fun and Engaging**

    - **Advice**: Make mind mapping enjoyable by using colors, images, and creative elements. Keeping it fun will increase your motivation to do it regularly.
    - **Example**: Use colored pens, stickers, or digital icons to make your mind maps visually appealing and engaging.

Setting Realistic Goals and Celebrating Progress

1. **Set Small, Achievable Goals**

    - **Advice**: Start with small, manageable goals to build confidence and momentum. Gradually increase the complexity and scope as you become more comfortable.
    - **Example**: Begin by mind mapping your daily tasks. Once you're consistent with that, move on to planning projects or setting long-term goals.

2. **Track Your Progress**

    - **Advice**: Keep track of your mind mapping activities to monitor your progress and identify areas for improvement.
    - **Example**: Maintain a journal or digital log of your mind maps. Review it weekly to see how you're progressing and make any necessary adjustments.

3. **Celebrate Milestones**

    - **Advice**: Celebrate your achievements, no matter how small. Recognizing your progress will keep you motivated and reinforce the habit.
    - **Example**: Treat yourself to something enjoyable when you reach a mind mapping milestone, such as completing a project plan or maintaining a daily mind mapping habit for a month.

4. **Reflect on the Benefits**

    - **Advice**: Regularly reflect on how mind mapping has positively impacted your life. This reflection can reinforce the habit and keep you motivated.

- **Example**: Take a few minutes each week to journal about the benefits you've experienced from mind mapping, such as improved organization, reduced stress, or better time management.

5. **Adjust and Adapt**
    - **Advice**: Be flexible and willing to adjust your approach as needed. If something isn't working, try a different strategy or tool.
    - **Example**: If you find it difficult to stick to a daily mind mapping routine, try switching to a weekly session or incorporating mind mapping into a different part of your day.

Example: Setting Realistic Goals and Celebrating Progress

1. **Initial Goal**: Create a daily mind map for one week.
    - **Steps**:
        - Set a daily reminder.
        - Spend 10 minutes each morning creating a mind map for the day's tasks.

- Track your progress in a journal.

2. **Progress Check**: After one week, review your journal to see how consistent you were and note any challenges or successes.

3. **Next Goal**: Expand to planning a small project using mind maps.

    - **Steps**:
        - Choose a simple project, such as planning a family outing or organizing a workspace.
        - Create a mind map to outline the project's steps and timeline.
        - Review and update the mind map regularly.

4. **Celebration**: At the end of the project, celebrate your accomplishment. Treat yourself to something enjoyable, like a favorite snack or a relaxing activity.

5. **Reflection**: Reflect on how mind mapping helped you with the project. Note any improvements in organization, clarity, or stress levels.

By following these strategies and setting realistic goals, you can develop a consistent mind mapping habit that enhances your ability to manage tasks, projects, and goals effectively. Remember, the key to success is persistence and adaptability. Celebrate your progress, learn from your experiences, and continue to refine your mind mapping practice.

Conclusion

Recap and Encouragement

As we reach the conclusion of this journey, let's take a moment to reflect on the key takeaways from "Mind Mapping for Women with Adult ADHD: Harnessing Your Brain's Full Potential and Empowering Your ADHD Journey." This book has provided you with a comprehensive understanding of mind mapping and its profound impact on managing ADHD.

We began by exploring the unique challenges faced by women with ADHD and the transformative power of self-acceptance and self-awareness. We delved into the concept of mind mapping, tracing its history and uncovering its numerous benefits. From understanding the science behind mind mapping and how it engages the ADHD brain to learning about various tools and techniques, you've gained valuable insights into how to effectively incorporate mind mapping into your life.

In the chapters that followed, we examined practical applications of mind mapping across different areas of your life—personal, professional, academic, and self-care. You've learned how to manage daily routines, organize tasks and projects at work, enhance creativity, improve time management, and plan self-care routines.

We also highlighted real-life success stories and personal testimonies to inspire and motivate you.

As you embark on your own mind mapping journey, remember that the process is unique to you. Embrace your creativity, be patient with yourself, and celebrate every milestone, no matter how small. The skills you've acquired will empower you to navigate the complexities of ADHD and harness your brain's full potential.

Words of Encouragement and Empowerment

Your journey with ADHD is one of resilience, strength, and endless potential. Mind mapping is a powerful tool that can help you unlock your creativity, improve your organization, and achieve your goals. It's a testament to your ability to adapt and thrive despite the challenges you face.

Believe in yourself and your capabilities. You have the power to transform your life and turn your dreams into reality. Every mind map you create is a step towards a more organized, focused, and fulfilling life. Embrace the journey, celebrate your progress, and continue to learn and grow.

Looking Forward

As you continue your journey with mind mapping, keep exploring, experimenting, and refining your techniques. There's always more to learn and discover. The resources and communities mentioned in this book are there to support you, provide inspiration, and connect you with others who share your journey.

I encourage you to share your experiences and stories. Your unique insights and achievements can inspire others and contribute to a growing community of women who are empowering themselves through mind mapping. Whether it's through online forums, social media groups, or local meetups, your voice matters and can make a difference.

In closing, remember that you are not alone on this journey. You are part of a vibrant, supportive community of women who are navigating the challenges of ADHD with courage and determination. Keep mind mapping, stay motivated, and continue to harness your brain's full potential. Your journey is just beginning, and the possibilities are limitless.

Thank you for embarking on this journey with me. I look forward to hearing about your successes and seeing the incredible mind maps you create. Together, we can empower each other and make our ADHD journeys a source of strength and inspiration.

www.ingramcontent.com/pod-product-compliance
Lightning Source LLC
Chambersburg PA
CBHW071928210526
45479CB00002B/595